I0413698

Nutrition Basics
For Your Good Health

© Copyright by Anna Douglas Madden
Author and Publisher
First Edition, May 18, 2016

A Grandmother's Pearls Publication
Douglas & Company Unlimited

Post Office Box 400469
Hesperia, California 92340
Telephone: 760-995-4963

The information contained within this material is true and accurate to be best of the publisher's knowledge at the time of printing. Every effort has been made for accuracy, but that is not always possible. No contents are intended to advertise or support any names, brands, products, goods, or services.

I would like to thank, in advance, everyone who provides feedback and sup-portive assistance for distribution of the project ❖

❧❧ Introduction ❧❧

THIS NUTRITION-RELATED MATERIAL was not compiled by the medical community, nor by a dietitian or nutrition expert, but rather, by a kind of "Doctor Gran" someone who wants to help sort out some of the madness and neglect surrounding nutrition issues of the day with a common-sense perspective *(in much the same way as our mothers and grandmothers use to do back in the good old days).*

"*Professionals*" have not done this for us. Although research studies are constantly conducted and volumes of information about foods and other nutrients are readily available in the marketplace, Americans are not *educated* about these subjects nor their health-related conditions.

As one writer indicated, when our bodies malfunction and we seek help, we're diagnosed with a *disease*, and it's matched with a corresponding pharmaceutical drug. If we can't be diagnosed, we're often labeled as depressed and given an anti-depressant. Then, we're referred from specialist to specialist: gastroenterologists, endocrinologists and rheumatologists, and given more drugs, namely immune-suppressants or steroid therapy. In reality, this resolves nothing and sets us up for much greater problems.

Also, we're over-exposed to commercialized claims about vitamins, minerals, anti-oxidants, gluten-free products, exercise equipment, treatments, etc. Yet, I've never heard one word about the extreme importance of enzymes and the immune system nor the significance of acid-alkaline pH balance. No one has mentioned a "leaky gut" nor what that means. Even though a goodly amount of food-related data is available, too often it tends to be fragmented and is only accessed after searching here, there, and everywhere. More often than not, our learning is forced upon us when beginning to cope with a new physical condition.

It is clear, that when it comes to proper concepts and nutrition, we can use all the help we can get, because in American society today, we seem to be more concerned with our outward appearance than with the stability of our inner health. And in line with this thinking, we seem to have adopted some very twisted values. We are taught to hate obesity but more from a cosmetic perspec-

tive than anything else. We've become a nation of people operating on the misguided notion that our value as a person is based upon our physical appearance; consequently, we have the spawned the tragedy of people making themselves gravely ill and dying, as a result of anorexia and other eating disorders. For the sake of our own mental and physical health, we need to develop a more common-sense approach than that.

We concern ourselves a lot about the cosmetics of being fat, but while it is fine not to want to be obese, the truth is that we need to be focused on making ourselves healthier by developing better eating habits, having more physical activity in our lives, and in most cases, a more sleek physique will probably be the welcome byproduct.

These materials were designed some years ago to be a quick-reference for the common types of nutrients we're ignorant about and those that can easily destroy us, because we consume them excessively. Too much fat not only makes us obese, but it can clog our arteries, leading to strokes, heart disease, and death. High cholesterol puts us at major risk of a heart attack, and too much sodium destroys kidneys and raises blood pressure *(causing hypertension)*—also a major risk determinant for heart attack and death.

It is a sad—and alarming—fact that we are wrecking our own health and that of our offspring with poor food choices. In the past, many of the high fat-cholesterol-sodium-sweet foods that use to be eaten only occasionally, have now become mainstays in many Americans' daily diets, i.e., fast foods, candies, desserts, and other highly processed foods that have no nutritive value. This is particularly bad for our children whose bodies most need good nutrition on which to build for a lifetime of service.

This basic nutritional material contains a variety of nutrient-health-related information which it is hoped you will find convenient and useful in your pursuit of establishing, or maintaining, the best possible health. The one thing not included in the main portions of the material pertains to gluten intolerance, but since it is an important issue of the day, the appendix section contains some information on the subject❖

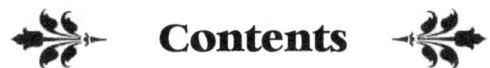

Contents

	PAGE
Basic Nutrition	1
FOOD COMPOSITIONS:	
Food Components	2
Vitamins	3-4
Minerals	5
Daily Nutrient Allowances	6
Vitamin Interactions	7
Essential Health Facts	8, 30
Fat Intake	9
Low Cholesterol Nutrition	10
Salt and Sodium Compounds	11
High Sodium Foods	12
Anti-oxidants and Free Radicals	12
Sugar and Sweeteners	13
Understanding Bottled Water	14
Microwave Safety	14
The Significance of Enzymes	15
FOOD EFFECTS:	
Food Digestive System	16
Food Combining for Health	17
Food Functions	18
Food that Matches Body Parts	19
Fiber-rich Foods	20-22
Acid-Forming and Alkalinizing Foods	23
Inflammation Causing and Inflammation Fighting Foods	24
Nightshade Vegetables and Fruits	25
FOOD & HEALTH:	
Chicken Wings Health Risk	25
Understanding Arthritis	26
Eczema Causes and Triggers	27
What is Diabetes?	28
Autoimmune Diseases	29
Essential Health Facts	30
APPENDIX:	
Codes and Abbreviations	32
Food Label Glossary	33
Serving Sizes Based on Hand	34
Measurements	35-36
Food Equivalents	37
What is Gluten?	38
Legume Intolerance	38
Food Handling Safety Tips	39
Index	40

Basic Nutrition Facts

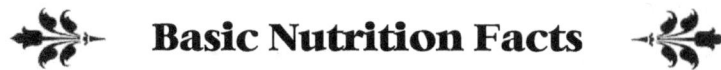

In the foods we eat, there are three main sources of calories: FATS, PROTEIN, and CARBOHY-DRATES. Most foods are a combination of at least two of these substances, and often include all three. The other components in our foods—vitamins, minerals, water, additives, etc., contribute only negligible, or no calories for energy.

The following list shows which food items fall under what category. Note that FATS have more calories per unit than either CARBOHYDRATES or PROTEIN in other words, fat is the most calorie-dense *(contains the most concentrated source of calories)* of all our foods. The government has established guidelines for the consumption of nutrients in each of these food categories.

FAT SOURCES *(9 calories per gram)*	CARBOHYDRATE SOURCES *(4 calories per gram)*	HIGH PROTEIN SOURCES *(4 calories per gram)*
Avocados	Breads and Rolls	Cheese
Bacon and Salt Pork	Cakes	Eggs
Baked Products	Candies	Fish and Seafood
Butter and Margarine	Cereals and Grains	Meats *(lean beef, lamb, pork, etc.)*
Cocoa Butter	Cookies and Crackers	Milk and milk products
Coconuts	Corn Meal	Poultry
Coffee Creamer	Dried Beans and Peas	Soy Products
Cream and half-n-half	Flour	Yogurt
Cheese	Fruit *(all)*	
Gravies	Pasta *(noodles, spaghetti, etc)*	
Ice Cream	Pastries	
Lard and Shortening	Popcorn	
Mayonnaise and Salad Dressings	Pretzels	
Meats *(marbled, or untrimmed)*	Potatoes	
Milk and Milk Products	Rice	
Nuts and Seeds	Sugars, Syrups, Jams, Jellies	
Oils *(All types)*	Sweet Potatoes	
Olives	Tortillas	
Peanuts and Peanut butter	Vegetables *(all)*	
Sauces	Yams	
Skin of Meat and Poultry		
Sour Cream		
Vegetables and Plants		

Note: Protein foods can vary greatly in how much FAT they also contain.
These items are classified into Lean, Medium-Fat and High-Fat groups.

 # Food Component Daily Allowances
(U.S. Food and Drug Administration)

NUTRIENT NAME	MAXIMUM DAILY VALUE (AMOUNT)	NUTRIENT FUNCTION
Total Fat	65 grams (g) *(or maximum 30-35% total calories)*	Provides energy, transports fat-soluble vitamins, helps form cell membranes and harmones
Saturated Fatty Acids	20 grams (g)	The basic chemical units in fat-may be either monounsaturated," or "polyunsaturated."
Cholesterol	300 milligrams (mg)	Needed to form hormones, cell membranes, and other body substances.
Sodium	2,300 milligrams (mg)	A mineral. Attracts water into the blood vessels and helps maintain normal blood volume and blood pressure. Needed for the normal function of nerves and muscles.
Total Carbohydrates	300 grams (g) *(or 50-55% of total calories)*	Includes starches, sugars, and dietary fiber. Starch and sugar supply energy to the body.
Fiber	25 grams (g)	Dietary fiber provides bulk which promotes regular elimination of body wastes.
Potassium *(an electrolyte)*	3,500 milligrams (mg)	Helps maintain body fluids.
Protein*	50 grams (g) *(or 5% of total calories)*	Forms the hormones and enzymes used to regulate body processes. Building blocks of the body. Needed for growth, maintenance, and replacement of body cells.
Water	6-8 glasses per day	Helps transport nutrients, removes body wastes, regulates body temperature, replaces water lost in urine and perspiration.

Please note: The daily value amounts are based upon a 2,000 calorie diet. A person's daily values may be higher or lower depending upon calorie needs. Also, the values for protein do not apply to certain populations; for these groups, nutrition experts of the Food and Drug Administration recommend the following:

Children 1 to 4 years:	16g
Infants less than 1 year:	14g
Pregnant women:	60g
Nursing mothers:	65g

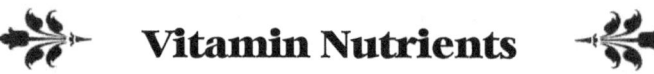

Vitamin Nutrients

Fat Soluble: *Stored in the body; toxicity (poisonous level) can result if excessive amounts are consumed*

SUBSTANCE NAME	FUNCTIONS	SOURCE
Vitamin A	Body tissue reparation and maintenance, vision *(necessary for night vision).*	Green & yellow fruits, vegetables, milk products, fish liver oil.
Vitamin D	Calcium and phosphorus metabolism *(bone formation)*, heart action, nervous system maintenance, normal blood clotting, skin reparation.	Egg yolks, organ meats, bone meal, sunlight, liver, milk, tuna/salmon *(canned)*
Vitamin E *(Tocopherol)*	Aging retardation, anti-clotting factor, blood cholesterol reduction, blood flow to heart, capillary wall strengthening, fertility, male potency, lung protection *(anti-pollution)*, muscle and nerve maintenance.	Dark green vegetables, eggs, liver, organ meats, wheat germ, vegetable oils, desiccated liver, oatmeal, peanuts, tomatoes.
Vitamin K	Essential in blood clotting.	Vegetables, body's own supply.

Water Soluble: *Excreted in the urine when the body receives excessive amounts.*

SUBSTANCE NAME	FUNCTIONS	SOURCE
Vitamin B1 *(Thiamin)*	Appetite, blood building, carbohydrates metabolism, circula-tion, digestion *(hydrochloric acid production)*, energy, growth, learning capacity, muscle tone mainte-nance *(intestines, stomach, heart).*	Black strap molas-ses, brewer's yeast, brown rice, fish, meat, nuts, organ meats, poultry, wheat germ, peanuts, sun-flower seeds, Brazil nuts.
Vitamin B2 *(Riboflavin)*	Antibody and red blood cell formation, cell respiration, metabolism *(carbohydrates, fat, protein).*	Black strap molas-ses, nuts, organ meats, whole grains, al-monds, Brus-sels sprouts, brewer's yeast, liver *(beef)*
Vitamin B6 (Pyridoxine)	Antibody formation, digestion *(hydrochloric acid pro-duction)*, fat and protein utilization *(weight control)*, maintains sodium/potassium balance *(nerves).*	Black strap molas-ses, brewer's yeast, green leafy vegeta-bles, meat, organ meats, wheat germ, whole grains, desic-cated liver, beef liver, prunes, brown rice, peas.

SUBSTANCE NAME	FUNCTIONS	SOURCE
Vitamin B12 (Cobalamin)	Appetite, blood cell formation, cell longevity, healthy nervous system, metabolism *(carbohydrate, fat, protein).*	Cheese, fish, milk, meat products, organ meats, cottage cheese, liver *(beef)*, tuna fish *(canned)*, eggs.
Vitamin B15 (Pangamic Acid	Cell oxidation and reparation, metabolism *(protein, fat, sugar)*, glandular and nervous system stimulation.	Brewer's yeast, brown rice, meat *(rare)*, seeds, *(sunflower, sesame, pumpkin)*, whole grains, meats.
Biotin (B Complex)	Cell growth, fatty acid production, metabolism *(carbohydrates, fat, protein)*, vitamin "B" utilization.	Legumes, whole grains, brewer's yeast, lentils, egg yolk, liver *(beef)*, soybeans.
Vitamin C	Forms substances that hold cells and the body together; Speeds the healing of wounds; Increases resistance to infection.	Citrus fruits, berries, cabbage, potatoes, vegetables.
Choline (B Complex)	Lecithin formation, liver and gall bladder regulation, metabolism *(fats, cholesterol)*, nerve transmission.	Brewer's yeast, legumes, organ meats, soybeans, wheat germ, lecithin, liver *(beef)*, egg yolks, peanuts.
Folic Acid (Folacin, Folate) (B Complex)	Appetite, body growth and reproduction, hydrochloric acid production, protein metabolism, red blood cell formation.	Green leafy vegetables, milk pro-ducts, organ meats, oysters, salmon, whole grains, brewer's yeast, dates *(dried)*, spinach, tuna fish *(canned)*.
Inositol (B Complex)	Retardation of artery hardening, cholesterol reduction, hair growth, lecithin formation, metabolism *(fat and cholesterol)*.	Black strap molasses, citrus fruits, brewer's yeast, dates *(dried)*, meat, milk, nuts, vegetables, whole grains, peanuts.
Niacin (Nicotinic Acid, Niacinamide) (B Complex)	Promotes healthy skin, nerves, and digestive tract; Also involved in use of body energy; Can help lower LDL *("bad cholesterol")* and triglycerides; Can help raise HDL *("good cholesterol")*.	Brewer's yeast, seafood, lean meats, milk products, poul-try, desiccated liver, rhu-barb, peanuts
Panto-Acid (Pantothenic Acid)	Antibody formation, carbohydrates, fat protein conversion *(energy)*, growth stimulation vitamin utilization.	Brewer's yeast, organ meats, salmon, wheat germ, whole grains, liver *(beef)*, mushrooms, elder-berries, orange juice.
PABA (Para Aminobenzoic Acid)	Blood cell formation, graying hair *(color restoration)*, intestinal bacteria activity, protein metabolism.	Black strap molasses, brewer's yeast organ meats, wheat germ.

Mineral Nutrients

Minerals in general, are required for body building and regulatory functions

SUBSTANCE NAME	FUNCTIONS	SOURCE
Calcium	Bone and tooth formation, blood clotting, heart rhythm, nerve tranquilization, nerve transmission, muscle growth & contrac-tion.	Milk, yogurt, other dairy products, molasses, bone meal
Chromium	Blood sugar level, glucose metabolism *(energy)*.	Brewer's yeast, clams, corn oil, whole grain cereals.
Copper	Bone formation, hair and skin color, hearing, processes of body hemoglobin and red blood cell formation.	Legumes, nuts, or-gan meats, seafood, rai-sins, molasses, bone meal.
Iodine	Helps regulate body energy, prevent goiter formation, aids mental development.	Table salt, milk, seafoods, kelp.
Iron	Hemoglobin development *(substance in red blood cells)*, facili-tates oxygen transportation throughout body.	Black strap molas-ses, eggs, fish, organ meats, poultry, wheat germ , desiccated liver, nuts, green vegetables
Magnesium	Aids in metabolism, assists in function of nerve and muscle fi-bers.	Bran, honey, green vegetables, nuts, seafood, spinach, bone meal, kelp tabs, peanuts, tuna (can)
Manganese	Enzyme activation, reproduction and growth, sex harmone production, tissue respiration, vitamin B1 metabolism, vita-min E utilization.	Bananas, bran, celery, cereals, leafy vegetables, legumes, liver, nuts, pineap-ples, whole grains
Phosphorus	Bone and tooth formation, cell growth and repair, energy pro-duction, heart muscle contraction, kidney function, me-tabolism *(calcium, sugar)*, nerve and muscle activity, vitamin utilization.	Eggs, fish, grains, glandular meats, poultry, yellow cheese.
Potassium	Heartbeat, rapid growth, muscle contraction, nerve tranquili-za-tion.	Dates, figs, peaches, tomatoes juice, black-strap molasses, nuts, raisins, sea-food.
Sodium	Normal cellular fluid, proper muscle contraction.	Salt, milk, cheese, seafood.
Sulfur	Collagen synthesis and body tissue formation.	Bran, cheese, clams, eggs, nuts, fish, wheat germ.
Zinc	Burn and wound healing, carbohydrate digestion, prostrate gland function, reproductive organ development and growth, metabolism of vitamin B1, Phosphorus, and protein.	Brewer's yeast, liver, seafood, soybeans, spinach, sunflower seeds, mushrooms.

Vitamin & Mineral Daily Allowance
(U.S. Food and Drug Administration)

Daily Reference Values (DRV)

FOOD COMPONENT	DAILY AMOUNT	MEASURE
Total Fat	65	grams (g)
Saturated fatty acids	20	grams (g)
Cholesterol	300	milligrams (mg)
Sodium	2300	milligrams (mg)
Potassium	3500	milligrams (mg)
Total carbohydrate	300	grams (g)
Fiber	25	grams (g)
Protein	50	grams (g)

Based on a 2000 Calorie Intake; for Adults and Children 4 or More Years of Age

Daily Reference Intake (DRI)

VITAMINS & MINERALS	DAILY AMOUNT	MEASURE
Vitamin A	5000	International Unit (IU)
Vitamin C	60	milligrams (mg)
Calcium	1000	milligrams (mg)
Iron	18	milligrams (mg)
Vitamin D	400	International Unit (IU)
Vitamin E	30	International Unit (IU)
Vitamin K	80	micrograms (µg)
Thiamin	1.5	milligrams (mg)
Riboflavin	1.7	milligrams (mg)
Niacin	20	milligrams (mg)
Vitamin B6	2.0	milligrams (mg)
Folate	400	micrograms (µg)
Vitamin B12	6.0	micrograms (µg)
Biotin	300	micrograms (µg)
Pantothenic acid	10	milligrams (mg)
Phosphorus	1000	milligrams (mg)
Iodine	150	micrograms (µg)
Magnesium	400	milligrams (mg)
Zinc	15	milligrams (mg)
Selenium	70	micrograms (µg)
Copper	2.0	milligrams (mg)
Manganese	2.0	milligrams (mg)
Chromium	120	micrograms (µg)
Molybdenum	75	micrograms (µg)
Chloride	3400	milligrams (mg)

Check with a qualified medical professional to determine if these are the appropriate nutrient amounts for you to take based upon your age and other factors.

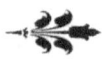

Vitamin Interactions with Drugs and Other Substances

SUBSTANCE NAME OR CATEGORY	AFFECT ON VITAMIN
Antacids	Interferes with vitamin C
Antibiotics	Interferes with most of the vitamin B group. Also Interferes with vitamin K.
Anticoagulants	Vitamin E alters patient's response; interferes with vitamins C and K.
Anticonvulsants	Interferes with vitamin D
Antidepressants	Interferes with vitamin C
Anti-diabetic Agents *(Oral)*	Vitamin C can magnify their effects; may interfere with vitamin B12.
Anti-hypertensives	Vitamin E can alter patient's response
Aspirin and Aspirin Substitutes	Interferes with vitamins K, B12, and C
Baking Soda	Interferes with vitamin B1
Chloramphenicol	Interferes with vitamin B12
Codeine	Interferes with vitamin B12
Contraceptives *(Oral)*	Interferes with vitamins C, E, B1, B2
Cortisone and prednisone	Interferes with vitamin C, vitamin B6, vitamin D
Diuretics	Interferes with vitamin C
Hydralazine	Interferes with vitamin B6
Indomethacin	Interferes with vitamin C
Iron	Interferes with vitamin E when taken with iron; Vitamin C enhances iron absorption.
Isoniazid *(INH)*	Interferes with vitamin B6
Methotrexate	Interferes with folic acid
Methlbromide *(preservative)*	Interferes with panthothenic acid
Mineral Oil	Interferes with fat-soluble vitamins A, E, K
Neomycin	Interferes with vitamin B12
Penicillamine	Interferes with vitamin B6
*Rancid *(decomposed, rank)* Oils and Fats	Can interfere with vitamin E
Soy / Soybeans	Interferes with Iodine
Steroids *(hormones)*	Interferes with vitamin C
Thyroid Hormones	Interferes with vitamin E

Fats and oils are used as "foods" and as "carriers" for medicines.

Do You Know These Essential Health Facts?

Recommended Levels

Blood Pressure	Less than 140/190
Total Cholesterol	100-199
HDL	39 or greater
LDL	0-99
VLDL	5-40
Triglycerides	0-149
Glucose (blood sugar)	Less than 100
Sodium Chloride	Less than 2,000 mg / day (World Health Organization)

Honey—a natural sweetener—is one of the only foods known to contain all the nutrients needed to sustain life.

Nutrient Blockers

➤ Intake of any kind of sugar weakens the immune system and has the potential to reduce the body's defenses against viruses and bacteria by 75% (or more) for four to six hours.

➤ Sugar destroys vitamin C in the foods we consume and other nutrients needed to combat illnesses.

➤ High sugar and high sodium (table salt) intake robs the body of calcium which can weaken bones and cause osteoporosis.

➤ Soybeans and soy products inhibit iodine—an essential mineral.

➤ Antibiotics interferes with most of the vitamin B group.

➤ Steroids, diuretics, and antacids block vitamin C.

SUGARS IN THE BEVERAGES PEOPLE DRINK & GIVE THEIR CHILDREN

NATURAL SUGARS (NUTRIENTS & SUGARS)

Item	Size / 4 oz	Amount	Size / 8 oz	Amount
Whole Milk	½ Cup	1.5 tsp	1 Cup	3 tsp
100% Orange Juice	½ Cup	2.5 tsp	1 Cup	5 tsp
100% Apple Juice	½ Cup	3 tsp	1 Cup	6 tsp
100% Grape Juice	½ Cup	4 tsp	1 Cup	8 tsp

= ¼ Cup sugar

ADDED SUGARS, CALORIES & MAN-MADE SUGARS

Item	Size / 4 oz	Amount	Size / 8 oz	Amount
Gatorade	½ Cup	1.5 tsp	1 Cup	3 tsp
Pepsi	½ Cup	2 tsp	1 Cup	4 tsp
Sunny Delight	½ Cup	2.5 tsp	1 Cup	5 tsp

= 1/8 Cup sugar

Note: An ordinary-sized (12 oz) can of Pepsi Cola soda pop contains 8 teaspoons of sugar. High fructose corn sugar is used in pop and has no nutritive value (no vitamins or minerals). A 12 oz Coca Cola contains 9.3 teaspoons of sugar. The American Heart Association recommends a maximum daily allowance of 6 teaspoons of sugar (25 grams, 100 calories) per day for women and 9 teaspoons for men (38 grams, 150 calories). Less for children who tend to be more hypersensitive.

Fat Intake and Food Facts

Substance Name	Daily Allowance	Nutrient Sources
Cholesterol	300 milligrams, or less, per day	A fat-like substance found in meat and organ meats, poultry, fish, milk, dairy products, egg yolks.
Monounsaturated fatty acids	Approximately 10 to 15 percent of total calories	Plants and animals, olives, peanuts, margarine, hydro-genated vegetable shorten-ings, etc.
Polyunsaturated fatty acids	Up to 10 percent of calories	Large portions found in fats from plants and vegetables, also in some fish.
Saturated fatty acids	8 to 10 percent of calories	Largest portions found in meat, poultry, dairy products and some vegetable oils, coconut oil, palm oil, palm kernal oil.
Total fat	30 percent or less of total calories	Meat, poultry, dairy products, plants, vegetables, etc.

❖❖ Nutrition Details ❖❖

Calories. Fats contain 9 calories per gram and all fats, regardless of their source, contain approximately the same number of calories.

Cholesterol. Most meats have about the same amount of cholesterol—roughly 70 milligrams per 3-ounce cooked serving. Shrimp and crayfish have more cholesterol than most other types of fish, but they are lower in total fat and saturated fatty acids than most meats and poultry. Egg yolks have a high cholesterol content *(200+ milligrams)*, therefore, consumption should be limited to 2-3 times per week.

The organ meats of animals *(liver, sweetbreads, kidneys, etc.)* are very high in cholesterol. Eat them only occasionally. Also avoid eating the skin of poultry and other animals.

Hydrogenated Fat. During food processing, fats may undergo a process known as hydrogenation. In margarine, this process allows an oil to be partly hardened and molded into tub or stick form. Recent studies suggest that these fats may raise blood cholesterol; therefore, these fats should only be used if they contain no more than two grams of saturated fatty acids per tablespoon.

High Fat Foods. Some prepared foods that are high in fat content include those that are fried, basted, au gratin, crispy, escalloped, pan-fried, sautéed, stewed, or stuffed. Cream sauces and dishes that are buttered, creamed, covered with cheese sauce or gravy, in hollandaise sauce, marinated, or in casseroles also tend to be high in fat.

Processed meats *(sausage, bologna, salami and hot dogs)* are high in calories and saturated fat. About 70-80 percent of their calories are derived from fat.

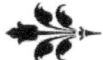 # Low Cholesterol Nutrition

FOODS RECOMMENDED	FOODS TO AVOID
Beverages • Coffee *(decaffeinated only)* • Citrus fruit juices *(at least 8 ounces daily)* • Vegetable juices • Milk *(fat-free only)*	**Beverages** • Coffee with caffeine • Cream • Chocolate-flavored beverages • Eggnog • While milk, whole-dried milk • Malted milk
Breads • Any bread not made with egg yolk, dried egg, lard, butter or cream.	**Breads** • All bread products containing egg yolk, dried egg, lard, butter or cream.
Cereals • Low-fat cereals eaten with skim milk.	**Cereals** • Cereals with high fat content.
Desserts • Fresh or cooked fruits • Jello • Angel food cake • Fruit pies made with egg white and liquid shortening. • Puddings made without egg yolk, or cream. • Sherbets	**Desserts** • Cakes, pies, desserts and puddings made with egg yolk, animal fats, dried egg, cream, cocoa, butter, or lard. • Ice cream
Fruits • At least 8 ounces of citrus fruit juices • Any fresh, frozen, cooked, or canned fruit.	
Meats, Poultry, Fish, Fats, Eggs, Cheese • Small servings of lean, broiled, roasted, or boiled beef, veal, lamb, or pork may be eaten occasionallyserved without gravy or sauces. • Chicken, or turkey *(lean, white meat without skin)*. • Fresh fish • Cottage cheese • Egg whites only • Margarine *(if not hydrogenated)* • Liquid vegetable oils *(corn, cottonseed, safflower, or soybean)*.	**Meats, Poultry, Fish, Fats, Eggs, Cheese** • Animal fats • Butter and hydrogenated margerines • Bacon, duck, mutton • Brains, liver, kidney • Crab meat, lobster, oysters, shrimp • Egg yolks and foods prepared with egg • Fish canned in oil • Lard • Stews, gravies, sauces prepared with fat • Sweetbreads
Soups • Vegetable soups made with skim milk and without meat stock.	**Soups** • Cream, meat stock, or chicken soups.
Vegetables • Fresh or frozen vegetables • Raw or cooked vegetables • Vegetables prepared in salads	**Vegetables** • Creamed, breaded, or fried vegetables
Miscellaneous • French dressing made with corn oil • Jam, jelly • Popcorn *(unbuttered)* • Rice (brown) • Spices, salt, vinegar	**Miscellaneous** • Buttered popcorn • Mayonnaise • Noodles • Nuts • White sauce

SUBSTANCE NAME	FUNCTION
Salt *Sodium Chloride):*	Used in cooking or at the table; also used in canning and pre-serving food products.
Baking Powder:	Used to leaven quick breads and cakes.
Baking Soda *(Sodium Bicarbonate):*	Used to leaven breads and cakes and sometimes added to vege-tables; also used as an alkalize for indigestion.
Disodium Phosphate:	Present in some quick-cooking cereals and processed cheeses.
Monosodium Gluta-mate (MSG):	A flavor enhancer/seasoner used in home, restaurant, and hotel cooking and in many packaged, canned and frozen foods.
Sodium Alginate:	Used in many chocolate milks and ice creams to make a smooth mixture.
Sodium Benzoate:	A preservative used in many condiments such as relishes, sauces, and salad dressings.
Sodium Caseinate:	A thickening and binding agent.
Sodium Citrate:	A buffer, used to control acidity in soft drinks and fruit drinks.
Sodium Hydroxide:	Used in processing to soften and loosen skins of ripe olives and certain fruits and vegetables.
Sodium Nitrate:	A curing agent for meats and sausages used to provide color and to prevent botulism *(food poisoning).*
Sodium Phosphate:	An emulsifier, stabilizer, and buffer.
Sodium Propionate:	A mold inhibitor used in pasteurized cheese and in some breads and cakes.
Sodium Saccharin:	An artificial sweetener.
Sodium Sulfite:	Used to bleach certain fruits such as maraschino cherries and glazed or crystallized fruits that are to be artificially colored; also used as a preservative in some dried fruits such as prunes.
Salt-Sodium Conversions:	¼ teaspoon salt = 500 milligrams sodium ½ teaspoon salt = 1,000 milligrams sodium ¾ teaspoon salt = 1,500 milligrams sodium 1 teaspoon salt = 2,000 milligrams sodium

❖❖ Nutrition Facts ❖❖

The human body requires only about 0.5 grams of salt, or 0.20 grams of sodium per day. The government's 2015 dietary guidelines recommend a daily intake allowance of less than 2,300 milligrams (2.3) grams per day.

It should also be noted that some over-the counter drugs contain large amounts of sodium. Antacids may also contain sodium. Check ingredient labels to verify content.

 # High Sodium Foods

Food Category	Food Name
Bread Products	• Salted crackers, pretzels, popcorn, potato chips • Commercially baked goods: cakes, cookies, pies, pastries, doughnuts, sweet rolls
Dairy Products	• Cheeses; buttermilk; Dutch process cocoa; instant cocoa mixes
Main Dish Items	• Pizza, lasagna, manicotti, ravioli, macaroni and cheese, cheese rarebit, cheese blintzes, quiche, soufflés • Canned or dehydrated soups or chowders • Commercially prepared main course foods: hash, stew, chili, meat pie, goulash, TV dinners or other frozen main dishes • Tacos, enchiladas, tamales, burritos, tostadas
Meat, Poultry, Fish	• Cured meats: ham, bacon, Canadian bacon, corned beef, luncheon meats (bologna, salami, turkey loaf, smoked beef, etc.) • Canned shellfish: shrimp, crab, clams, oysters, scallops, lobster • Fish: commercially frozen, pre-breaded, pre-fried, smoked • Frankfurters: wieners, hot dogs, etc. • Sausages: Breakfast-type or substitutes, Polish, Italian, Mexican
Meat Substitutes	• Salted nuts or seeds; canned beans and peas; soy protein products
Vegetable Products	• Canned and frozen vegetables and vegetable juice.
Miscellaneous	• Catsup, chili sauce • Mayonnaise, commercial and packaged salad dressings • Meat tenderizer, monosodium glutamate (MSG) • Olives, pickles, pickle relish • Salted gravies and sauces (barbecue, soy, steak, Worcestershire, smoke-flavored sauces) • Seasoning salts: garlic, onion, celery, etc.

 ## Antioxidants and Free Radicals

ANTIOXIDANTS ARE NUTRIENTS that fight and defeat destructive cells—free radicals. Bodies make some antioxidants and some are traditionally supplied in the diet (fruits, vegetables). However, environmental influences have increased the need for antioxidants beyond what they are capable of producing, and even beyond diet. The three major antioxidant vitamins are beta-carotene, vitamin C, and vitamin E.

You'll find them in colorful fruits and vegetables – especially those with purple, blue, red, orange, and yellow hues. For optimal health and immune functioning, people should eat the recommended dietary allowance (RDA) of antioxidant vitamins and minerals to stay healthy and avoid deficiencies. Note that when taking supplements, moderation is very important, because the fat soluble vitamins (A, D, E, K) are stored in the body and eliminated slowly—getting too much can be toxic.

Oxygen is the basis for the formation of free radicals. Human bodies require large amounts of it for metabolism, which is breaking down nutrients for energy—for every function.

Additional free radicals can be caused by *environmental sources* like tobacco smoke, oil fumes, chemicals, pollutants, radiation, the sun or ozone. Disease creates free radicals, and so does exercise. Free radicals cause cell mutations, damage immune function, cause wrinkles and aging and are a contributing cause behind many diseases. Free radical proliferation can also be caused by a lack of *antioxidants* in the diet, or the inability of the body to produce enough of them.

Sugar & Sweeteners

CATEGORY	DESCRIPTION
Primary Sugar Sources	cornstarch, grapes, honey, maple trees, milk sugar, sugar beets, sugar cane, other foods.
Chemical Makeup of Sugars	• blackstrap.low grade molasses used .....for animal food • brown sugar .... refined for home use • corn syrup .... derived from corn starch • dextrose ... .derived from dried glucose • fructose ....also called 'levulose' • glucose..........syrupy liquid combination used in confectionery, alcohol fermentation, tanning, and treating tobacco • honey ....contains glucose & fructose • Lactose ....a by-product of cheese processing • Maltose ....small amounts occur in cereals, legumes • molasses.. .... residue from sugar-refining process • Nutrisweet ....sugar substitute, artificial sweetener • raw sugar. .... 97-99% sucrose • saccharin.. ....sugar substitute, artificial sweetener • sucrose......... .... .refined sugars for home use (white granulated, powdered, etc.)
Food Category of Sugar	carbohydrate, highest energy substance
Uses of Sugar in Food	*baked* goods candies and chocolates canned fruits, jams, jellies, marmalades chewing gum enhance taste and smell of fruits frozen foods soft drinks sweetener for other foods and beverages
Drug Uses of Sugar	disguise bitter taste
Caloric Properties of Sugar *(granulated, white)*	1 *teaspoon* ....= 15 calories 1 tablespoon = 45 calories 1 ounce = 109 calories 1 cup = 774 calories

❖❖ Nutrient Facts ❖❖

The major health risks of excessive sugar intake is that it may trigger the onset of diabetes mellitus and consuming too much sugar also contributes to tooth decay.

Some people like to use Agave nectar (pronounced 'uhGAHvay'), because they believe it is a naturally occurring sweetener; however it is not. This nectar is a highly processed syrup made from the Agave tequiliana (tequila) plant that is stripped of all nutritional value. It is about 1-1/2 times sweeter than regular sugar and contains roughly 60 calories per tablespoon. The end product contains more fructose than HFCS, which reportedly makes it extremely dangerous to consume!

Understanding Bottled Water

SUBJECT	MEANING
Artesian Well Water:	Water drawn from a well where the aquifer *(a water-bearing rock formation)* is above the level of the natural water table.
Distilled Water:	Water that has been vaporized and then condensed to remove minerals.
Mineral Water:	Water collected at a borehole or spring or spring originating from a geologically and physically protected underground water source.
Purified Water:	Water that has been either distilled, deionized, or passed through membrane filters to remove particles in a process called "reverse osmosis.
Spring Water:	Water collected as it flows naturally to the surface from a spring or from a borehole to the underground source of the spring.
Well Water:	Water collected from a hole drilled to tap an aquifer.

❖❖ Nutrient Facts ❖❖

Carbonated water, soda water, tonic water, and seltzer water are considered soft drinks and are regulated separately from other bottled waters.

❖❖ Food-Related Fact - Safe Use of Microwave Ovens ❖❖

Low-frequency EM (electromagnetic) radiation is emitted by a typical microwave oven; reportedly, it is often intense and extensive. (e.g. 40 mG at 60 cm). Therefore, it is recommended that individuals keep at least 1.5 meters (5 feet) away from a microwave oven while it is in use.

The Significance of Enzymes

ENZYMES REPRESENT THE FOOD-DIGESTING BIOCHEMISTRY of the body involving the mouth, throat, stomach, pancreas, liver and intestines (see chart on page 16). It is extremely important to understand that enzymes are specialized food components, and a different one is required to digest every nutrient—solid food, beverage, or spice. Specific enzymes work on specific foods; the right type of enzyme is needed for the food to be chemically broken down. Undigested, and partially digested, foods are responsible for many autoimmune diseases, because their toxicity can leak into the blood system.

Listed below are the common enzyme categories and the food types they act upon.

Digestive enzymes are enzymes that break down food into usable material. The major different types of digestive enzymes are:

amylase – breaks down carbohydrates, starches, and sugars which are prevalent in potatoes, fruits, vegetables, and many snack foods:

- lactase – breaks down lactose (milk sugars);
- diastase – digests vegetable starch;
- sucrase – digests complex sugars and starches;
- maltase – digests disaccharides to monosaccharides (malt sugars);
- invertase – breaks down sucrose (table sugar);
- glucoamylase – breaks down starch to glucose;
- alpha-glactosidase– facilitates digestion of beans, legumes, seeds, roots, soy products, and underground stems.

protease – breaks down proteins found in meats, nuts, eggs, and cheese:

- pepsin – breaks down proteins into peptides;
- peptidase – breaks down small peptide proteins to amino acids;
- trypsin – derived from animal pancreas, breaks down proteins;
- alpha – chymotrypsin, an animal-derived enzyme, breaks down proteins;
- bromelain – derived from pineapple, breaks down a broad spectrum of proteins, has anti -inflammatory properties, effective over very wide pH range;
- papain – derived from raw papaya, broad range of substrates and pH, works well breaking down small and large proteins.

lipase – breaks down fats found in most dairy products, nuts, oils, and meat.

cellulase – breaks down cellulose, plant fiber; not found in humans.

❖❖ Timing ❖❖

Enzymes work on contact, so they must be in physical contact with a food or substance in order to be effective. Enzymes that are not produced by the body usually come in capsules that can be opened or swallowed, or as enterically coated tablets. Capsules are preferable because they can either dissolve in the stomach releasing the enzymes, or the capsules can be opened and the enzymes mixed with any food or drink and taken at the beginning of a meal. This allows the enzymes to be breaking down food in the stomach before passing into the small intestine.

Since liquid leaves the stomach first, It is important not to consume beverages 30 minutes prior to a meal because enzymes will go away with it causing unresolved food conditions.

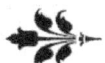 

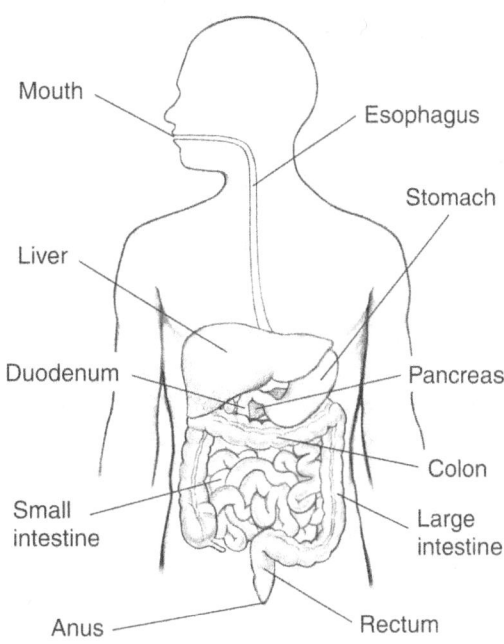

Mouth	The mouth is the beginning of the digestive tract. Chewing breaks food down into pieces for digestion while saliva helps mix it into a form the body can absorb and use.
Esophagus	The esophagus receives swallowed food and delivers it with muscular contractions into the stomach.
Stomach	It holds food while it is being mixed with hydrochloric acid and enzymes and then releases it into the small intestine.
Liver	It secrets bile into the small intestine and detoxifies potentially harmful agents. The liver is the body's chemical "factory." It processes raw materials absorbed by the small intestine and makes all the various chemicals the body needs to function.
Pancreas	The pancreas secretes digestive enzymes into the small intestine. It also makes and places insulin in the bloodstream to metabolize sugar.
Gallbladder	It concentrates and stores bile that it releases into the small intestine to help absorb and digest fats.
Small Intestine	A 22-foot long muscular tube that breaks down food using enzymes released by the pancreas and bile from the liver for the absorption of nutrients into the bloodstream. Leftover-food then moves on to the large intestine (colon).
Colon (Large Intestine)	The colon is a 6-foot long tube that connects the small intestine to the rectum. It processes waste (mostly food debris and bacteria) left over from the digestive process and empties it into the rectum once or twice a day to begin the process of eliminating unneeded materials from the body.
Rectum	It is an 8-inch chamber that connects the colon to the anus and receives stool (waste) from the colon and holds it until evacuation.
Anus	The anus is the last part of the digestive tract. It is a 2-inch canal that holds stool from the rectum until its contents are released into a toilet, or elsewhere.

Food Combing for Health

FOOD COMBINING is based upon the idea that meals, and snacking, should be kept simple to properly digest food the natural way wherein the body can work to break down food and absorb nutrients within appropriate timeframes. Proper food combining can result in improved metabolism and weight loss.

Since different foods require their own unique enzymes and time lengths, too many provisions in one meal confuse the digestive system, and it can't produce all of the required enzymes. No enzymes—no digestion. Also, foods, and beverages, with no nutritive value can not be properly digested. This leads to a multitude of issues that may include heartburn, intestinal gas, abdominal pain, inflammation, destructive free radical cells, unrecognized foodstuff stored as fat, etc. These consistent practices will ultimately lead to far more serious consequences and may cause irreversible harm.

Many issues arise when the wrong foods are eaten together or enzymes aren't available and food can't be appropriately digested; that causes a toxic body. In those situations, food can't be broken down into parts that the body can assimilate (use). Undigested food eventually leaves the stomach, many times, small portions get into the intestinal tract, become trapped in crevices, and putrefy. Inflammation and overworked organs are the result and lead to malfunctions of various kinds—a toxic blood stream, allergic reactions, and a variety of sicknesses and diseases.

General Combining Rules

Eat protein with vegetables only
Eat vegetables with starches OR protein
Legumes may be combined with proteins, starches, grains
Oil and fats combine with all foods
(but slows the digestive process)

NEVER combine protein with starches
NEVER mix starches and sugar
NEVER combine sweet fruits with other foods
NEVER combine melons with other foods

Melons should be eaten only with other melons
apples with apples
berries with berries
citrus with citrus
pears with pears
grapes alone
Acid fruits and sub-acid fruits may be combined

Fruit should be eaten alone and only in the mornings until noon--on an empty stomach.

NEVER DRINK WHILE EATING!!
Exception: 1/2 cup water to take vitamins, minerals, and/or enzymes with meal
Drink water, or other liquids, no less than one hour before and/or no less than one and a half hours after meals.

Food Digestion Timeframes

Water	15 Minutes
Melons	1 Hour
Fruit	1-2 Hours
Vegetables	2-5 Hours
Fat	3 Hours
Starch	3 Hours
Protein	4 + Hours

Fruit and sweet foods have relatively "simple" carbohydrate structures—meaning they digest very quickly.

When eaten with other foods, sweets break down first, while other foods sit in the stomach and ferment. Therefore, it is best to eat dessert first (at least 30 minutes before a meal) or at least 4 hours afterwards.

Grazing (eating on top of undigested food) should also be avoided, because it too causes fermentation and gastro issues.

Food Functions

Vegetables with Diuretic Effect
(They flush fluid from the body)

Artichokes
Asparagus
Beets
Cabbage
Carrots
Celery
Cucumbers
*Eggplant
Fennel
Lettuce
Onions and garlic
Parsley
Pumpkin
Tomatoes (actually a fruit)
Watercress

*Some people have trouble digesting eggplants; use carefully.

Fruits with Diuretic Effect
(They flush fluid from the body)

Apples
Bananas
Black currants
Blackberries
Blueberries
Coconuts
Cranberries
Figs
Grapefruit
Grapes
Juniper berries
Kiwi
Lemons
Mango
Papaya
Peaches
Pears
Pineapple
Raspberries
Strawberries

MELONS

Cantaloupe
Honeydew melon
Watermelon
(one of the very best diuretic fruits)

Healing Herbs and Spices

Black Pepper	Helps relieve indigestion
Cinnamon	Helps lower blood pressure
Clove	Anti-microbial
Dill	Treat heartburn, colic and gas
Fennel	Can reduce bad breath and body odor
Fenugreek	Helps flush out harmful toxins
Garlic	Natural antiseptic
Ginger	Anti-nausea remedy
Mint	Can ease hiccups
Oregano	Helps soothe stomach muscles
Rosemary	Antioxidant
Sage	Antiseptic and antibiotic
Thyme	Relaxes respiratory muscles
Turmeric	Anti-cancer

Vegetable by Colors to Eat for Health

White	To strengthen the immune system.
Yellow	To fortify skin elasticity.
Orange	To prevent inflammation
Red	To improve heart blood health
Purple	To protect the nervous system
Green	To detoxify.

Kidney Cleanser

Take a bunch of parsley or Cilantro (Coriander Leaves) and wash it clean. Cut it into small pieces and put it in a pot and pour in clean water. Boil for ten minutes and let it cool down, then filter it and pour in a clean bottle. Keep inside refrigerator to cool.

Drink one glass daily and notice that all salt, and other accumulated poison, come out kidney by urination.

Use sparingly, as these vegetables can be very potent.

Foods That Match Body Parts

These are foods that resemble, and provide nutrients to many parts of the human body. According to nutritionists, most of these foods are more beneficial when eaten raw.

Food Name	Looks Like...
Avocados and Pears	*Female womb and cervix.* When women eat one avocado a week, it balances birth hormones and can prevent cervical cancer.
Banana	*Facial smile.* When digested, converts into a neurotransmitter called serotonin, which is a mood regulating chemical in the brain.
Broccoli	*Cancer cells.* Team of researchers at US National Cancer Institute found that weekly serving of broccoli reduced risk of prostate cancer by 45%.
Carrot	*Human eye.* Increases blood flow to the eyes. Orange color is from a plant chemical called *betacarotene*, which reduces risk of developing cataracts.
Celery, Rhubarb, Bok-choy	*Bones structure.* Human bones are 23% sodium, and so is celery. These vegetables all provide sodium - without it, bones are weak.
Clams	*Testicles.* Supplementing diets with folic acid and zinc—both of which clams are high in - can have a significant effect on improving semen quality in men.
Figs	*Male sperm.* Figs are full of seeds and hang in twos. Studies show that Figs increase sperm count and help overcome male sterility.
Ginger	*Stomach.* Aids in digestion, calms stomach, cures nausea, and motion sickness. Also slows down the growth rate of bowel tumors.
Grapefruits, Oranges, Other Citrus Fruits	*Mammary glands of the female.* Assists in health of the breasts and the movement of lymph in and out of them. Grapefruit contain limonoids, which helps inhibit the development of cancer.
Grapes	*Lungs.* Fresh grapes help reduce risk of lung cancer and emphysema. Grape seeds can help reduce the severity of asthma triggered by allergy.
Kidney Beans	*Human kidneys.* These beans are shaped like them and actually heal and help maintain kidney function.
Mushrooms	*Human ear.* When sliced in half, resembles the shape of the mushroom. Improves hearing abilities, since they contain Vitamin D.
Olives	*Women's ovaries.* Italian study found that women whose diets included a lot of olive oil had a 30% lower risk of ovarian cancer.
Onions	Human body's cells. Onions clear waste materials from all body cells. They also produce tears which wash the epithelial layers of the eyes.
Red wine	*Blood.* Rich in antioxidants and polyphenols. Contains a blood-thinning compound that reduces blood clots associated with stroke and heart disease.
Sweet Potatoes	*Pancreas.* Can balance the glycemic index of diabetics. High in beta-carotene - a potent antioxidant that protects all tissues of the body.
Tomato	*Heart.* The tomato has four chambers and is red in color, so also does the human the heart. Tomatoes are loaded with lycopine, which is a perfect heart and blood nutrient.
Walnut	*Brain - Left and right hemisphere.* Helps in developing over three dozen neuron-transmitter links between brain cells in the human brain.

Fiber-Rich Foods

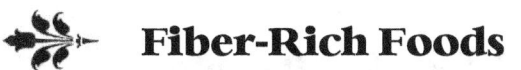

Bran	Portion	Amount of Fiber
All Bran Cereal	1/2 cup	10 g
Corn bran, raw	1 ounce	22 g
Fiber One Bran Cereal	1/2 cup	14 g
Oat bran, raw	1 ounce	12 g
Rice bran, raw	1 ounce	6 g
Wheat bran, raw	1 ounce	12 g

Whole Grains	Portion	Amount of Fiber
Barley, pearled, cooked	1 cup	6 g
Bread (whole wheat), sliced	1 slice	2 g
Brown rice, cooked	1 cup	4 g
Buckwheat groats, cooked	1 cup	5 g
Bulgur, cooked	1 cup	8 g
Crackers, rye wafers	1 ounce	6 g
Millet, cooked	1 cup	2 g
Oats (old fashioned), dry	1/2 cup	4 g
Popcorn, air popped	3 cups	4 g
Rye flour, dry	1/4 cup	7 g
Spaghetti (whole wheat), cooked	1 cup	6 g
Wheat berries, dry	1/4 cup	5 g
Wheat flour (whole wheat), dry	1/4 cup	4 g
Wild rice, cooked	1 cup	3 g

Beans	Portion	Amount of Fiber
Adzuki beans	1 cup	17 g
Black beans	1 cup	15 g
Broad beans (fava)	1 cup	9 g
French beans	1 cup	17 g
Garbanzo beans	1 cup	12 g
Kidney beans	1 cup	16 g
Lentils	1 cup	16 g
Lima beans	1 cup	14 g
Navy beans	1 cup	19 g
Pinto beans	1 cup	15 g
White beans, small	1 cup	19 g
Yellow beans	1 cup	18 g

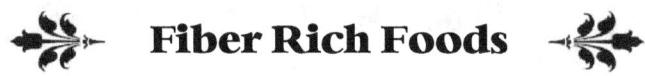

Fiber Rich Foods

Peas	Portion	Amount of Fiber
Cow peas (blackeyes), cooked	1 cup	11 g
Peas (edible podded), cooked	1 cup	5 g
Peas, green, frozen	1 cup	14 g
Peas, split, cooked	1 cup	16 g
Pigeon peas, cooked	1 cup	9 g

Berries	Portion	Amount of Fiber
Blackberries, raw	1 cup	8 g
Blueberries, raw	1 cup	4 g
Boysenberries, frozen	1 cup	7 g
Currants (red and white), raw	1 cup	5 g
Elderberries, raw	1 cup	10 g
Gooseberries, raw	1 cup	6 g
Loganberries, frozen	1 cup	8 g
Raspberries, raw	1 cup	8 g
Strawberries, raw	1 cup	3 g

Vegetables	Portion	Amount of Fiber
Beet greens	1 cup	4 g
Broccoli, cooked	1 cup	5 g
Brussels sprouts, cooked	1 cup	6 g
Collard greens	1 cup	5 g
Kale, cooked	1 cup	3 g
Mustard greens	1 cup	5 g
Red cabbage, cooked	1 cup	4 g
Savoy cabbage, cooked	1 cup	4 g
Spinach	1 cup	4 g
Swiss chard	1 cup	4 g
Turnip greens	1 cup	5 g
Cauliflower, cooked	1 cup	5 g
Kohlrabi raw	1 cup	5 g

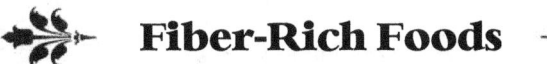

Squash (Cooked)	Portion	Amount of Fiber
Acorn squash	1 cup	9 g
Crookneck squash	1 cup	3 g
Hubbard squash	1 cup	7 g
Spaghetti squash	1 cup	2 g
Summer scallop squash	1 cup	5 g

Hot Potatoes (Cooked)	Portion	Amount of Fiber
Russet potato, flesh and skin	1 medium	4 g
Red potato, flesh and skin	1 medium	3 g
Sweet potato, flesh and skin	1 medium	4 g

Fruit	Portion	Amount of Fiber
Banana	1 medium	3 g
Pear	1 medium	6 g
Orange	1 medium	4 g
Apple	1 medium	4 g
Prunes, dried	½ cup	6 g
Raisins	2 ounces	2 g
Peaches, dried	1/4 cup	3 g
Figs, dried	1/2 cup	8 g
Avocado, raw	1/2 fruit	9 g

Nuts and Seeds	Portion	Amount of Fiber
Almonds	1 ounce	4 g
Brazil nuts	1 ounce	2 g
Cashews	1 ounce	1 g
Flaxseed	1 ounce	8 g
Peanuts	1 ounce	2 g
Pinon nuts	1 ounce	12 g
Pistachio nuts	1 ounce	3 g
Pumpkin seeds	1/2 cup	3 g
Sesame seeds	1/4 cup	4 g
Sunflower seeds	1/4 cup	3 g
Walnuts	1 ounce	2 g

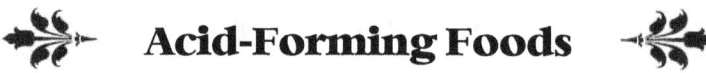

Acid-Forming Foods

OVER-ACIDITY IN THE BODY comes from consuming too many acid-forming foods and not enough alkalizing foods. Below is a brief list of acidic foods that can throw off the body's pH system and the alkaline foods that help restore and maintain balance.

Adzuki Beans
Alcoholic drinks
Artificial Sweeteners
Barley Syrup
Beef
Beet Sugar
Black Beans
Blueberries
Bran
Brazil nuts
Breads and grain products
Cane Sugar
Cashews
Cereals - hot or cold
Cheese - Parmesan & sharper varieties
Chicken
Coconut - dried
Coffee, other caffeinated drinks
Colas
Cornmeal
Crackers
Cranberries

Filbert Nuts
Fish
Fructose
Garbanzo Beans
Honey – Processed
Ketchup - unless natural & home-made
Lactose
Lamb
Lentil Beans
Macadamia Nuts
Maple Syrup
Mayonnaise - unless natural & homemade
Molasses
Mustard - powder and processed
Navy Beans
Nutmeg
Oats
Other Beans – unless sprouted
Pastas
Pastries
Peanuts

Pecans
Pinto Beans
Pistachio Nuts
Plums
Popcorn
Pork
Prunes
Pumpkin Seeds
Red Beans
Rice
Rye
Soy Sauce
Spelt
Sunflower Seeds
Table Salt - Refined
Tobacco
Vinegar
Walnuts
Wheat
Wheat germ
Yogurt - sweetened

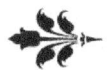 # Alkalinizing Foods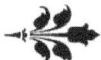

Alfalfa
Almonds
Amaranth
Arrowroot Flour
Brewer's Yeast
Brown Rice Syrup
Butter - fresh unsalted
Cayenne Pepper
Chestnuts
Chia sprouted seeds
Coconut - fresh
Cream
Dried Sugar Cane Juice (Sucanat),
Eggs

Flax
Fruit Juice
Fruits - most
Garlic
Gelatin
Green/Snap Beans
Herbal Teas - most
Herbs - most
Honey - raw, unpasteurized
Lima Beans
Margarine
Milk - including goat's
Millet
Miso
Oils: cold-processed

Peas
Pignoli Nuts
Potatoes
Quinoa
Radishes
Sea Salt - unprocessed
Sesame - unsprouted
Soybeans
Spices - most
String Beans
Vanilla Extract
Vegetable Juices - all
Vegetables - most
Whey
Yogurt - plain

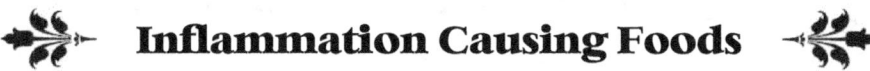

Inflammation Causing Foods

MANY ORDINARY FOODS IN NORTH AMERICAN DIETS cause (or intensify) irritation in the body, and now most chronic conditions like cancer, arthritis, diabetes, and obesity are linked to inflammation conditions. In world-wide studies, the following list has been found to be primary factors:

- **Hydrogenated and trans-fats** (margarine, shortening, lard, oils and products commercially-made with them).

- **Meat (not wild-caught fish)** (injected with hormones and antibiotics; raised on genetically altered foods).

- **Fried foods** (French fries, chips, onion rings, nachos, hamburgers, chicken and chicken wings, etc.).

- **White sugar and sweets** (includes soft drinks and sweetened juices, baked goods). Addictive and leaches (sucks) calcium from bones.

- **Synthetic sweeteners** (Nutrasweet, Splenda, saccharin, aspartame, Amino-Sweet, etc.)

- **Iodized Salt** (lacks natural minerals)

- **Food additives**: (colors, flavor enhancers, stabilizers, preservatives, etc.)

- **Dairy products** (milk, yogurt, ice cream, cottage cheese, butter, processed cheese, etc.).

- **Wheat products** (genetically modified, unnatural).

- **Other gluten-containing grains**.

- **Alcohol** (High in sugar and a burden on the liver and skeletal system).

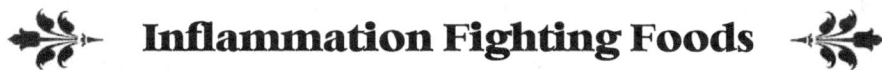

Inflammation Fighting Foods

Blackberries
Blueberries
Raspberries
Strawberries
Cayenne Pepper
Celery & Celery Seeds
Cherries
Black Cherries
Dark Green Vegetables
Fish
Flax seeds and Flax Oil
Ginger
Turmeric
Walnuts (unsalted)

THESE FOODS BELONG TO THE FAMILY OF SOLANACEAE PLANTS—a species of provisions that is inedible for some people, because of causing one or more of the following miserable effects: inflammatory painful joints associated with arthritis, gas, bloating, diarrhea, nausea, headaches and/or depression.

- **Potatoes:** This includes white, red, yellow and blue-skinned potato varieties; however, sweet potatoes and yams are not nightshades.

- **Peppers:** All peppers are in the nightshade family. This includes bell peppers (green, yellow, red), jalapenos, habaneros, cayenne peppers and paprika—a spice made from ground, dried peppers; however, peppercorns are not included in the group.

- **Eggplant:** All varieties of eggplant are nightshade vegetables that are commonly featured in Italian, Thai, East Indian and other ethnic cuisines.

- **Tomatoes:** Scientifically, this food's category is fruit because of its seeds. It is available in a variety of forms including tomato sauced, ketchup, soups, condiments, salsas, hot sauces, marinades and other forms for food preparation and consumption.

- **Tomatillos:** These nightshade fruits grow in warm climates and can be found as a wild weed in parts of Mexico. When ripe, they're either pale yellow or purple with a slight citrus-like flavor. Tomatillos are often featured in sauces and salsas.

- **Goji:** These small, slightly sweet red (wolfberries) are native to Asia. They're consumed raw, dried or made into juice (but are also sometimes ingredients in smoothies, teas and nutritional supplements).

Other berries that are nightshades include garden huckleberries, ground cherries and cape gooseberries. However, not normal gooseberries or blueberries.

Nightshade foodstuffs are used in a variety of cuisines; therefore, be sure to read labels thoroughly. Also, communicate well with people who prepare foods to be eaten so that no negative effects will be experienced.

❖❖ Chicken Wing Health Risk ❖❖
(An Internet Posting)

Avoid eating chicken wings frequently - ladies, especially; a true story! A friend of mine recently had a growth in her womb and she underwent an operation to remove the cyst.

The cyst removed was filled with a dark colored blood. She thought that she would be recovered after the surgery but! she was terribly wrong. A relapse occurred just a few months later. Distressed , she rushed down to her gynecologist for a consultation.

During the meeting, her doctor asked her a question that puzzled her. He ask if she was a frequent consumer of chicken wings and she replied yes wondering as to how, he knew of her eating habits. You see, the truth is in this modern day and age; chickens are injected with steroids to accelerate their growth so that the needs of this society can be met. This need is none other than the need for food. Chickens that are injected with steroids are usually given the shot at the neck or the wings.

Therefore, it is in these places that the highest concentration of steroids exists. These steroids have terrifying effects on the body as it accelerates growth. It has an even more dangerous effect in the presence of female hormones, this leads to women being more prone to the growth of a cyst in the womb❖

Understanding Arthritis

ARTHRITIS IS NOW THE LEADING DISEASE CAUSING DISABILITIES in the United States. It is NOT a single disorder—it is a generic term referring to joint pain and disease. There are more than 100 different **types of arthritis** and related conditions affecting individuals of every age and kind throughout the world. There is no know reason, but it impacts more females than males. Joint symptoms occur more frequently as people grow older.

The following is a list of the primary Arthritis categories:

Adult-onset Still's disease
Ankylosing Spondylitis
Back Pain
Behcet's Disease
Bursitis
Calcium Pyrophosphate Deposition Disease (CPPD)
Carpal Tunnel Syndrome
Chondromalacia Patella
Chronic Fatigue syndrome
Complex Regional Pain Syndrome
Cryopyrin-Associated Periodic Syndromes (CAPS)
Degenerative Disc Disease
Developmental-Dysplasia of Hip
Ehlers-Danlos
Familial Mediterranean Fever
Fibromyalgia
Fifth Disease
Giant Cell Arteritis
Gout
Hemochromatosis
Infectious Arthritis
Inflammatory Arthritis
Inflammatory Bowel Disease
Juvenile Arthritis
Juvenile Dermatomyositis (JD)
Juvenile Idiopathic Arthritis (JIA)
Juvenile Scleroderma
Kawasaki Disease
Lupus
Lupus in Children & Teens
Lyme Disease
Mixed Connective Tissue Disease

Myositis (inc.Polymyositis, Dermatomyositis)
Osteoarthritis
Osteoporosis
Pagets
Palindromic Rheumatism
Patellofemoral Pain Syndrome
Pediatric Rheumatic Disease
Pediatric SLE
Polymyalgia Rheumatica
Pseudogout
Psoriatic Arthritis
Reynaud's Phenomenon
Reactive Arthritis
Reflex Sympathetic Dystrophy
Reiter's Syndrome
Rheumatic Fever
Rheumatism
Rheumatoid Arthritis
Scleroderma
Sjögren's Disease
Spinal Stenosis
Spondyloarthritis
Systemic Juvenile Idiopathic Arthritis
Systemic Lupus Erythematosus
Systemic Lupus Erythematosus in Children & Teen
Systemic Sclerosis
Temporal Arteritis
Tendinitis
Vasculitis
Wegener's Granulomatosis

Eczema symptoms can be brought on by food and other factors. The exact causes of the disease is unknown. Sometimes people inherit a predisposition for eczema. They may have a family member who has eczema or who has hay fever or asthma. Many doctors think eczema causes are linked to allergic disease, such as hay fever or asthma. Up to 80% of children with eczema will develop hay fever and/or asthma.

There are many triggers of eczema that can make it flare-up or get worse. Below are some of the common ones. People should learn what causes their eczema to break out, and then try to avoid it.

Foods:

Atopic eczema can sometimes be caused by food allergens, especially before the age of one. Some studies of children and young people with atopic eczema found that one-third to nearly two-thirds also had a food allergy. Food allergies associated with eczema causes are typically:

➤ Dairy products
➤ Eggs
➤ Nuts and seeds
➤ Soy products
➤ Wheat

Allergens:

If genes make an individual more likely to develop atopic eczema, the condition will develop after they are exposed to certain environmental factors, such as allergens. They are substances that can cause the body to react abnormally. This is known as an allergic reaction. Some of the most common allergens that can be causes of eczema include:

➤ House dust mites
➤ Pets (cats & dogs)
➤ Pollens (seasonal)
➤ Molds
➤ Dandruff

Other Irritants:

These can make symptoms worse. However, what irritates one person may be different from what aggravates someone else with the same condition, but could include:

➤ Soaps and detergents
➤ Shampoos, dishwashing liquids
➤ Bubble Bath
➤ Disinfectants like chlorine
➤ Contact with juices from fresh fruits, meats, vegetables

Microbes:

Some types of microbe can be triggers of eczema:

➤ Certain bacteria like Staphylococcusaureus
➤ Viruses
➤ Certain Fungi

Stress:

Stress is known to be associated with eczema, but it is not fully understood how it affects the condition. Some people with eczema have worse symptoms when they are stressed. For others their eczema symptoms cause them to feel stressed.

Hormones:

Hormones are chemicals produced by the body. They can cause a wide variety of effects. When the levels of certain hormones in the body increase or decrease, some women can experience flare-ups of their eczema❖

❧ — What is diabetes? —❧

DIABETES IS A FOOD-RELEATED CONDITION affecting countless numbers of people. In the United States, it now claims more lives than AIDS and breast cancer combined. This disease takes 1 American every 3 minutes and is a leading cause of vision loss, heart disease, stroke, kidney failure, amputation of toes, feet or legs, and premature death. According to the Center for Disease Control, 29 million people in America (9.3 percent) have diabetes, and another 86 million adults aged 20 years and older have pre-diabetes.

Diabetes has everything to do with insulin in the body. Eaten food turn into sugars—or glucose. At that point, the pancreas organ should release insulin enabling it to open cells and allow the glucose to be used for energy. However, with diabetes, the system doesn't work, and several major things can go wrong—causing the onset of diabetes.

Kinds of Diabetes. Type 1 and type 2 diabetes are the most common forms of the disease, although there are other sorts, such as gestational diabetes, which occurs during pregnancy, as well as other forms.

Most Severe Diabetes. It is type 1—or insulin-dependent and sometimes called "juvenile" diabetes, because this disease usually develops in children and teenagers, although it can develop at other ages.

Immune System Malfunction. With type 1 diabetes, the body's immune system attacks part of the pancreas, when it mistakenly sees the insulin-producing cells in the organ as foreign, and destroys them. This attack is known as "autoimmune" disease. These islets cells (EYE-lets) are the ones that sense glucose in the blood, and in response, ordinarily produce insulin to normalize blood sugar levels.

Insulin is the key to open cells, allowing the glucose to enter and provide energy. However, without insulin—there is no "key."   So, the sugar stays and accumulates in the blood causing the body's cells to starve from the lack of glucose. When left untreated, the high level of "blood sugar" damage eyes, kidneys, nerves, and the heart, and can also lead to coma and death.

The most common form of diabetes is called type 2, or non-insulin dependent diabetes. This is also called "adult onset" diabetes, since it typically develops after age 35. However, a growing number of younger people are now developing type 2 diabetes.

People with the type 2 disease are able to produce some of their own insulin. However, often, it's not enough, and sometimes, the insulin will try to serve as the "key" to open the body's cells—but the key won't work—and the cells won't open; This is considered "insulin resistance".

Treatment. Often, type 2 diabetes results from being overweight and a sedentary lifestyle. Treatment involves improved diet and exercise. If blood sugar levels are still high, oral medications are used to help the body use its own insulin more efficiently. In some cases, insulin injections are necessary.

The CDC claim is that one in four people with diabetes doesn't know that he or she has it. How the organization arrives at that figure is unclear, but their 2014 records do show that Non-Hispanic black, Hispanic, and American Indian/Alaska Native adults are about twice as likely to be diagnosed with diabetes as non-Hispanic white adults. However, the latter group represents 35% of the pre-diabetes group❖

Autoimmune Diseases

THIS HAS TO DO WITH MALFUNCTIONS OF THE IMMUNE SYSTEM. It is very much impacted by nutrition intake. There are as many as 80 types of autoimmune diseases, and 75% affected are women. Genetic predisposition makes up about one third of the risk of developing an autoimmune disease, and the other two-thirds risks come from environmental factors that include: diet, lifestyle, infections (both prior and continual) exposure to toxins, hormones, excess weight, etc.

Autoimmune disease is caused by the immune system losing its ability to distinguish proteins belonging to a body with proteins belonging to foreign invaders. What causes symptoms is the buildup of damage to cells, tissues and/or organs in the body–damage caused by the immune system attacking those cells. Which proteins/cells are attacked is what separates one disease from another. The following are some of the more common autoimmune diseases:

Addison's Disease:	adrenal hormone insufficiency;
Celiac sprue Disease:	a reaction to gluten (found in wheat, rye, and barley) that causes damage to the lining of the small intestine;
Graves' Disease:	overactive thyroid gland;
Hashimoto's Disease:	inflammation of the thyroid gland;
Inflammatory Bowel Diseases:	a group of inflammatory diseases of the colon and small intestine;
Pernicious Anemia:	decrease in red blood cells caused by inability to absorb vitamin B12;
Psoriasis:	a skin condition that causes redness and irritation as well as thick, flaky, silver-white patches;
Reactive Arthritis:	inflammation of joints, urethra, and eyes; may cause sores on the skin and mucus membranes;
Rheumatoid Arthritis:	inflammation of joints and surrounding tissues;
Scleroderma:	a connective tissue disease that causes changes in skin, blood vessels, muscles, and internal organs;
Sjögren's Syndrome:	destroys the glands that produce tears and saliva causing dry eyes and mouth; may affect kidneys and lungs;
Systemic Lupus Erythematosus:	affects skin, joints, kidneys, brain, and other organs;
Type 1 Diabetes:	destruction of insulin producing cells in the pancreas;
Vitiligo:	white patches on the skin caused by loss of pigment.

Nutrition plays a strong role in autoimmune diseases, and while there are no cures, permanent remission can be achieved. An environment conducive to healing is created by addressing important lifestyle factors and changing dietary focus (if necessary) to eating nutrient-dense foods that provide all of the building blocks needed to resolve inflammation and support organ function—everything a body needs to properly regulate the immune system.

One of the most important contributors to autoimmune disease is nutrient deficiency. A leaky gut (comp-romised protective lining) is believed to be involved in all autoimmune diseases (and present in every autoimmune disease which has been tested). This is directly related to diet and lifestyle (the foods eaten, the foods not eaten, how much sleep and how much stress is in a person's lifestyle.

It is recommended that individuals with an autoimmune condition get plenty of rest, avoid stress and follow a strict diet free of inflammatory producers that include the list below and many other irritants:

> ➢ Nightshades Foods
> ➢ Fructose consumption in excess of 20g per day
> ➢ Non-nutritive (artificial) sweeteners
> ➢ NSAIDS (like aspirin or ibuprofen)
> ➢ Emulsifiers, thickeners, and other food additives
> ➢ Possibly dairy products

What is Blood Pressure?

Pressure of the blood on the walls of blood vessels and especially arteries.

Systolic (A Measurement)

The top number, which is the higher of the two numbers that measures the pressure in the arteries when the heart beats (when the heart muscle contracts).

Diastolic (A Measurement)

The bottom number, which is also the lower of the two numbers, measures the pressure in the arteries between heartbeats (when the heart muscle is resting between beats and refilling with blood).

Hypertension (High Blood Pressure)

Blood pressure is determined both by the amount of blood the heart pumps and the amount of resistance to blood flow in the arteries. The more blood the heart pumps and the narrower the arteries, the higher the blood pressure. High blood pressure is a common condition in which the long-term force of the blood against the artery walls is high enough that it may eventually cause health problems, such as heart disease.

What Causes a Stroke?

A stroke occurs when the blood supply to part of the brain is interrupted or severely reduced, depriving brain tissue of oxygen and nutrients. Within minutes, brain cells begin to die. Prompt treatment is crucial. Early action can minimize brain damage and potential complications.

What Causes a Heart Attack?

A heart attack occurs when the flow of blood to the heart is blocked, most often by a build-up of fat, cholesterol and other substances, which form a plaque in the arteries that feed the heart (coronary arteries). The interrupted blood flow can damage or destroy part of the heart muscle.

What is Diabetes?

There are two kinds:

> **Type 1** is a chronic condition in which the pancreas produces little or no insulin—a hormone needed to allow blood sugar (glucose) to enter cells to produce energy.

> **Type 2** diabetes occurs when the body becomes resistant to insulin or doesn't make enough insulin. It can sometimes be controlled by proper diet.

> **Hyperglycemia** is when there is not enough insulin in the body.

> **Hypoglycemia** is when blood sugar concentrations fall below normal.

What is Cholesterol?

Cholesterol is a lipid - which is a fatty, waxy necessary substance that is found in the cells of all animals and human beings. The body uses it to help build cells and produce hormones. Too much cholesterol in the blood can build up inside arteries, forming what is known as plaque. There are several kinds of cholesterol—primarily:

> **HDL (high density lipoprotein)** known as the "good cholesterol," picks up cholesterol from the blood and delivers it to cells that use it, or takes it back to the liver to be recycled or eliminated from the body.

> **LDL (low density lipoprotein)** carries mostly fat and only a small amount of protein from the liver to other parts of the body. Considered the "bad" cholesterol, because high levels can contribute to strokes, heart attacks, atherosclerosis, etc..

> **VLDL: (very low-density lipoprotein)** distributes the triglyceride produced by the liver.

> **Triglycerides (plasma lipids).** Any calories not used are changed into triglycerides and stored as fat for later use.

Who to contact regarding donation of body organs and transplants?

www.organdonar.gov

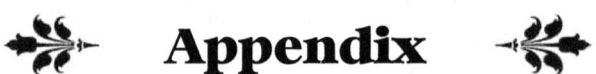 **Appendix**

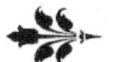 

<	= greater than
>	= less than
%	= percentage
--	= not available
Approx	= apprzoximately
Cal	= calories
Carbs	= carbohydrates
achol	= cholesterol
Diam	= diameter
Fl	= fluid
fl oz	= fluid ounce
Gal	= gallon
Gm	= gram
IU	= international units
lb(s)	= pound(s)
Lrg	= large-sized
Mcg	= microgram(s)
Med	= medium-sized
Mgs	= milligrams
Oz	= ounce
Pkg	= package
Pkt	= packet
Pt	= pint
Qt	= quart
Sm	= small-sized
Sod	= sodium
Tbsp	= tablespoon
Tsp	= teaspoon
Tr	= trace
w/	= with
w/o	= without

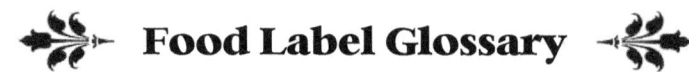

KEY WORDS	MEANINGS
Calorie Free	Less than 5 calories per serving
Fat Free	Less than 0.5 of fat per serving
Light *(Lite)*	⅓ less calories or no more than ½ the fat of the higher-calorie, higher-fat version or no more than ½ the sodium of the higher- sodium version
Reduced Fat	At least 25% less fat per serving than the higher-fat version
Low Fat	3 grams of fat (or less) per serving
Lean	Less than 10 grams of fat, 4 grams of saturated fat and 95 milligrams of cholesterol per serving
Extra Lean	Less than 5 grams of fat, 2 grams of saturated fat, and 95 milligrams of cholesterol per serving
Cholesterol Free	Less than 2 milligrams of cholesterol and 2 grams *(or less)* of saturated fat per serving
Low Cholesterol	20 milligrams of cholesterol *(or less)* and 2 grams of saturated fat *(or less)* per serving
Reduced Cholesterol	At least 25% less cholesterol than the higher-cholesterol version, and 2 grams *(or less)* of saturated fat per serving
Low in Saturated Fat	1 gram saturated fat *(or less)* per serving and not more than 15% of calories from saturated fatty acids
Sodium Free *(no sodium)*	Less than 5 milligrams of sodium per serving, and no sodium chloride *(NaCl)* in ingredients
Very Low Sodium	35 milligrams of sodium (or less) per serving
Low Sodium	140 milligrams of sodium (or less) per serving
Reduced or Less Sodium	At least 25% less sodium per serving than the higher-sodium version
Sugar Free	Less than 0.5 gram of sugar per serving
High Fiber	5 grams of fiber (or more) per serving
Good Source of Fiber	2.5 to 4.9 grams of fiber per serving of fiber per serving

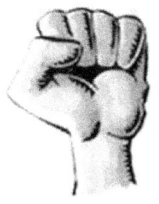

1 fist = 1 cup
*The size of fist also
= 1 medium-sized whole fruit*

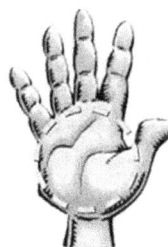

Palm = 3 oz.
meat, fish or poultry.
*(Sometimes equated to
the size of a deck of cards.)*

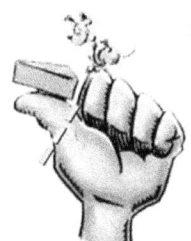

Thumb (tip of base)
= 1 oz of cheese

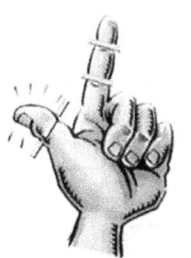

Index finger
(1st joint to 2nd joint) = 1 inch

Thumb tip = 1 teaspoon
3 teaspoons = 1 tablespoon

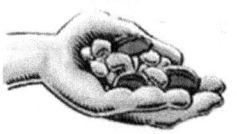

Palm = 3 oz. meant, fish
or poultry.
*(Sometimes equated to
the size of a deck of cards.)*

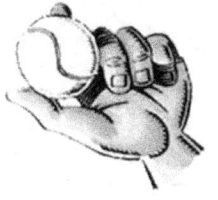

1 Tennis Ball
= 1/2 cup
1/2 of fist also = 1/2 cup

Measurements by Volume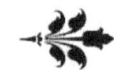

Pinch

Pinch or dash	= less than ⅛ teaspoon

Teaspoon

1 teaspoon	= ⅓ tablespoon	= ⅙ fluid ounce

Tablespoon

1 tablespoon	= 3 teaspoons	= ½ fluid ounce
2 tablespoons	= ⅛ cup	¹⁄₁₆ = pint	= 1 fluid ounce
4 tablespoons	= ¼ cup		= 2 fluid ounces
5⅓ tablespoons	= ⅓ cup		= 2.6 fluid ounces
8 tablespoons	= ½ cup		= 4 fluid ounces
10⅔ tablespoons	= ⅔ cup		= 5.3 fluid ounce
12 tablespoons	= ¾ cup		= 6 fluid ounces
16 tablespoon	= 1 cup	= ½ pint	= 8 fluid ounces

Cup

⅛ cup	= 2 tablespoons			= 1 fluid ounce
¼ cup	= 4 tablespoons			= 2 fluid ounces
⅓ cup	= 5⅓ tablespoons			= 2.6 fluid ounces
½ cup	= 8 tablespoons			= 4 fluid ounces
⅔ cup	= 10⅔ tablespoons			= 5.3 fluid ounces
¾ cup	= 12 tablespoons			= 6 fluid ounces
1 cup	= 16 tablespoons	= ½ pint		= 8 fluid ounces
2 cups	= 1 pint	= ½ quart		= 16 fluid ounces
4 cups	= 2 pints	= 1 quart		= 32 fluid ounces
8 cups	= 4 pints	= 2 quarts		= 64 fluid ounces
16 cups	= 8 pints	= 4 quarts	= 1 gallon	= 128 fluid ounces

Pint

½ pint	= 1 cup		= 8 fluid ounces
1 pint	= 2 cups		= 16 fluid ounces
2 pints	= 4 cups	= 1 quart	= 32 fluid ounces
4 pints	= 8 cups	= 2 quarts	= 64 fluid ounces
8 pints	= 16 cups	= 4 quarts	= 1 gallon	= 128 fluid ounces

 Measurements by Volume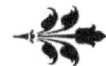

Quart				
½ quart	= 2 cups	= 1 pint		= 16 fluid ounces
1 quart	= 4 cups	= 2 pints		= 32 fluid ounces
2 quarts	= 8 cups	= 4 pints	= ½ gallon	= 64 fluid ounces
4 quarts	= 16 cups	= 8 pints	= 1 gallon	
8 quarts	= 32 cups	= 16 pints	= 2 gallons	= 1 peck

Measurements by Weight

1000 milligrams		= 1 gram
1 gram	= 0.035 ounce	
100 grams	= 3.57 ounces	
1 ounce		= 28.35 grams
½ pound	= 8 ounces	= 225.8 grams
1 pound	= 16 ounces	= 453.6 grams

Metric Measurements

1 milliliter		= 0.34 fl. ounces	
1 tablespoon	= 15 milliliters		
2 tablespoons	= 30 milliliters	= 1 fluid ounce	
1 cup	= 237 milliliters		
1 pint		= 0.47 liters	
1 liter		= 2.1 pints	= 1.06 qrt. = 0.26 gallons
1 quart	= 946 milliliters	= 0.95 liters	
1 gallon	= 3.8 milliliters	= 3.8 liters	= 4 quarts

Food Equivalents

Cheese and Eggs

1 pound process cheese shredded .... equals 4 cups
12 to 14 egg yolks .... equals 1 cup
8 to 10 egg whites .... equals 1 cup

Crumbs

20 saltine crackers .... yields 1 cup fine crumbs
12 graham crackers .... yields 1 cup fine crumbs
22 vanilla wafers .... yields 1 cup fine crumbs
8 to 9 slices zwieback .... yields 1 cup fine crumbs
1 slice bread .... yields ½ cup soft crumbs

Nuts

1 pound almonds in shell .... yields about 1 cup, shelled
1 pound walnuts in shell.. yields 2 cups, shelled
¼ pound chopped walnuts .... yields about 1 cup

Fruits and Vegetables

Grated peel of 1 lemon.. yields 1 teaspoon
Grated peel of 1 orange .... yields about 2 teaspoons
Juice of 1 lemon .... yields 3 to 4 tablespoons
Juice of 1 orange... yields 6 to 7 tablespoons
1 medium apple .... yields 1 cup chopped
1 medium onion .... yields ½ cup chopped
¼ pound celery *(about 2 stalks)* .... yields 1 cup chopped

Pasta and Grains

4 ounces uncooked macaroni *(1-1¼ cups)*............................. yields 2¼ cups cooked
4 ounces uncooked noodles *(1½-2 cups)*............................... yields 2¼ cups cooked
4 ounces uncooked spaghetti *(1-1¼ cups)*............................ yields 2½ cups cooked
1 cup uncooked rice *(6½ to 7 ounces)* .... yields 3-3½ cups cooked
1 cup precooked rice .... yields 2 cups cooked

What is Gluten?

ACCORDING TO THE CELIAC FOUNDATION, gluten is a general name for the proteins found in wheat, rye, barley and triticale. Gluten helps foods maintain their shape, acting as glue that holds food together. Gluten can be found in many types of foods and products—including some medications.

THE BIG 3 - WHEAT, BARLEY, RYE:

Wheat is commonly found in:
- breads
- baked goods
- soups
- pasta
- cereals
- sauces
- salad dressings
- roux

Barley is commonly found in:
- malt
- food coloring
- soups
- malt vinegar
- beer

Rye is commonly found in:
- rye bread, such as pumpernickel
- rye beer
- cereals

Triticale is a newer grain, specifically grown to have a similar quality as wheat, while being tolerant to a variety of growing conditions like rye. It can potentially be found in:
- breads
- pasta
- Cereals

Gluten intolerant people are now buying, or making, gluten-free products to eat. Fortunately, many supermarkets and other resources are beginning to carry them and also alternative grains and pre-mixed products. It is also very helpful that some restaurants are beginning to include gluten-free meals on their menus. It is recommended that people research their medications to ensure that they contain no gluten.

 # Legume Intolerance

MANY PEOPLE DON'T EAT BEANS, because they experience the misery and embarrassment of gas (flatulence). Although there are claims that beans can cause inflammatory conditions, for those who still would like to include them in their diet, some dietitians say the following actions will make it possible to eat beans: Cover them thoroughly with three times the water, and pre-soak the beans overnight. They'll double in size and most of the water will have been absorbed by morning. Rinse and drain the beans three or four times till the water runs clear. Cover in a pot and simmer until well done.

One person warned not to add salt to the beans while cooking them, indicating that salt prevents them being able to absorb the liquid they're cooked in. Adding a pinch of baking soda to the beans after they're done also helps to eliminate the gas-producing factor.

Food Handling Safety Tips

1. Bring groceries home and store them immediately after shopping.

2. Thoroughly wash hands in warm, soapy water before and after eating or handling food, after handling toxic products, pets, hair or plants, and after each use of the toilet.

3. Cleanse all dishes and other food-related items with soap and water each time they are used. Scrub counter tops and other areas where food is prepared.

4. Thoroughly wash raw fruits and vegetables before eating them.

5. Prevent cross-contamination between raw and cooked foods by using separate dishes; cutlery; cooking pots and pans; other tools; and preparation areas for them.

6. Refrigerate foods that will spoil at room temperatures, and refrigerate leftovers immediately after meals are finished.

7. Do not permit refrigerator, or freezer, doors to hang open when not in use.

8. Cook meats, poultry, fish and seafood until well done.

9. Keep highly perishable foods refrigerated, or on a bed of ice, until ready to serve or store.

10. Never drink from beverage containers that someone else has used, or will use.

11. Never eat directly from cooking pots or containers that hold food which others will eat.

12. Never eat from the dishes, silverware, or other containers that someone else has used, or will use.

13. Never feed children from the dishes, silverware, or beverage containers of others.

❖❖ Food Poisoning ❖❖

FOOD POISONING OCCURS when staphylococcus *(staph)* bacteria infect food, and these germs are capable of multiplying rapidly. Some foods are more easily contaminated by staph than others. These include mayonnaise *(and anything with mayonnaise in it);* cheeses and other dairy products which include sour cream; cream pies; and fish, meats, poultry and stuffings. Exercise special precautions when handling these foods.

Food poisoning symptoms include intestinal pain and cramps, nausea, vomiting and diarrhea. Some individuals experience profuse sweating or chills and overproduction of saliva. Shock may occur in serious cases. Symptoms usually appear abruptly within 2 to 4 hours of eating contaminated food, and they generally subside within 4 to 24 hours.

Note: E-Coli contamination occurs when food or water is exposed to urine or fecal bacteria. Since consumers don't know which purchased products may have been affected, scrubbing or appropriately cooking them will render risky foods safe to eat. E-Coli symptoms may be mild or severe, and similar to those described above; they may appear within 1 to 2 hours or up to a day later. When suspicious of contamina-tion exposure, seek immediate medical attention because a life could depend upon it❖

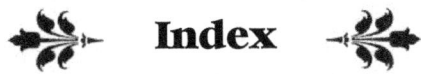

Index

Abbreviations and Codes   32
Acid-Forming Foods   23
Alkalinizing Foods   23
Anti-oxidants and Free Radicals   12
Appendix   31
Arthritis   26
Autoimmune Diseases   29
Basic Nutrition   1
Bottled Wate   14
Chicken Wings Health Risk   25
Codes and Abbreviations   32
Daily Nutrient Allowances   6
Diabetes   28
Eczema Causes and Triggers   27
Enzymes Significance   15
Fat Intake   9
Fiber-rich Foods   20-22
Food Combining for Health   17
Food Components   2
Food Digestive System   16
Food Equivalents   37
Food Functions   18
Food Handling Safety Tips   39
Food Label Glossary   33
Food that Matches Body Parts   19
Free Radicals and Anti-oxidants   12
Gluten   38
Health Facts, Essential   8, 30
High Sodium Foods   12
Index   40
Inflammation Causing Foods   24
Inflammation Fighting Foods   24
Legume Intolerance   38
Low Cholesterol Nutrition   10
Measurements   35-36
Microwave Safety   14
Minerals   5
Nightshade Fruits   25
Nightshade Vegetables   25
Salt and Sodium Compounds   11
Serving Sizes Based on Hand   34
Sugar and Sweeteners   13
Vitamin Interactions   7
Vitamins   3-4